ELVIS AND THE JOUR

THE PURPOSE O:

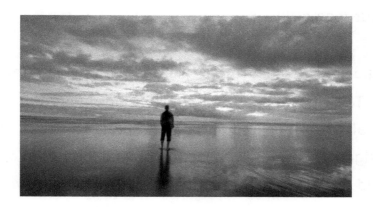

There once lived a young man named Elvis who was very curious about the meaning of life and wanted to know the purpose behind it all.

Daily these thoughts plagued his mind, in his sleep he had dreams where he searched for the meaning of life and during the day he had conversations where he hoped to glimpse the answers to his questions. But daily this strange truth of life seemed to elude him, so one day he picked up his bag and decided to say goodbye to his beautiful little house and go on the search for these answers.

"I have waited so long for life to bring me the answers and now I shall wait no more, I am done waiting, now I shall begin the search myself," Elvis said to himself as he carried his little bag and began this journey in search of the purpose of life.

He had journeyed a great distance when he came to a river. The river was sparkling white and beautiful flowers grew all around it like nature had blessed the river with a hedge. The river was peaceful and beautiful flowers floated steadily on its surface. Close your eyes and imagine this beautiful river, see the flowers all around the riverbank, see the flower petals floating, slow and steadily on the river, and listen to the wonderful songs of the fairies coming from the flowers and the chirping of the birds. The river looked, sounded, and scented like a paradise. But Elvis was very thirsty and did not pay attention to the strange singing coming from the flowers or the strange beauty of the river, he bent down and drank from the river, eager to quench his thirst. He drank for a while before he realized the singing had stopped and he looked up to find a crowd of tiny little fairies of various shapes and sizes all staring curiously at him as their tiny transparent wings flapped in the air.

"Who are you, young human? And what brings you to the land of fairies?" The largest of the fairies asked, he seemed like the leader.

"My name is Elvis and I am journeying in search of the meaning of life" Elvis answered, now squatting at the river bank.

"That is a noble journey indeed. One of great wisdom" The fairy said

"But tell me young human, what have you learned on your journey so far?" asked another fairy

Elvis thought for a while before answering "nothing in the least, I have not found any answers yet"

All the fairies were quiet for a while before the leader of the fairies nodded and said to Elvis "Come, maybe you can learn a thing or two from us"

Elvis jumped up eagerly and followed after the fairies, wondering if they could truly give him the answer he sought. He followed after the fairies wondering where it was that they were taking him.

They came to a point where a bush of thorns blocked their path, the leader of the fairies stretched forth his hands and the thorns disappeared to reveal a tiny little village, which was beautiful beyond what words could tell.

"This is our home," said the leader of the fairies, flying into the village with the other fairies, they flew in and out of the little houses in excitement.

"Life to us is about doing what we love, we can't work hard forever. For us, life is about enjoying nature, the sounds of birds, and each moment, that is the purpose of life for us" said the leader of the fairies.
Elvis pondered the fairy's words for a while and yet was not satisfied.
The fairies invited him to rest and stay with them for a few days, which he did and on the second day, Elvis picked up his bag, said thank you to the fairies, and continued his journey, he was still not satisfied with the answer he had gotten but he could not deny that he had learned a lot.

Elvis continued his journey and had walked for quite a while climbing mountains and traveling through rivers before he got to the great caves, where the cavemen lived.

They welcomed him eagerly because they had not seen any other human in ages.

"What brings you here, young human," The leader of the cavemen said that night as they ate roasted deer meat under the night sky. The stars twinkled and the moon glowed, the earth was beautiful and radiated such peace. If you close your eyes, you could hear the sounds of the crickets, see the starry night sky, the light from the moon as it illuminated the land, smell the wonder of nature in the air, smell the flowers, the trees, and all the beauty all around.

Close your eyes for a moment and picture the peacefulness of this moment, see the starry night, as the stars twinkled in the sky.

"I am on a journey to find the purpose of life," said Elvis and the cavemen gave him a nod of respect.

"That is a wise journey indeed, but tell me young man, what have you learned so far on this wonderful journey of yours?" The cavemen asked Elvis.

"I visited the fairies and they showed me great wisdom, they taught me that the beauty of life is in enjoying each moment and not about working hard forever. They say life is about enjoying, the birds, the air and nature all around" said Elvis as he munched on a piece of deer meat.

The cavemen listened to his words and looked at one another.

"Well, that is quite different from what we believe is the purpose of life" answered the cavemen.

"What do you believe is the purpose of life?" Elvis asked curiously.

"Look at our caves," the leader of the cavemen said pointing at the caves behind them, where the cavemen lived.

"We have spent years separating ourselves from other humans, we live alone, in peace, and enjoy nature. The beauty of life for us is to live secluded from the constant chaos of other humans and enjoy the peace of nature and be able to work hard to our satisfaction" the leader of the cavemen answered and Elvis pondered his words for a while utterly confused as to why anyone would be satisfied to live segregated from others of their kind.

"But don't you want to be free to meet others like you and enjoy life together, sharing and learning?" asked Elvis, confused by the way of life of the cavemen.

"No, to stay alone, away from the constant crowd and live life the way one wants is truly living" answered the caveman and Elvis could only stare in confusion.

He was not satisfied with this answer either and the next day he said thank you and goodbye to the cavemen and continued on his journey in search of the purpose of life.

Elvis journeyed on and on, going through forests, climbing great mountains, and passing through mighty rivers before he finally came to the land of the magicians. The streets were lined with magical carpets that took you all around the city. The magicians wore magnificent robes that had the image of the sun, moon, and stars drawn on them and the robes sparkled and glowed under the sun. The city was a wonder to behold.

Elvis rode on a magical carpet and looked in awe at the city, as he watched from the skies.

The city was amazing, it seemed like a dream. He had been riding for a long while before he decides to settle in front of a magnificent building that held such splendor and wonder.

The carpet dropped Elvis at the door and Elvis straightened his clothes before knocking boldly a the door.

A very tall magician, with lots of gray hair on his head, opened the door, the magician looked wise beyond his years and Elvis was sure he would have the answers to the purpose of life.

"Hello, young man, don't stand out there in the cold, come in and seat, have some tea, it's been ages since I had a visitor who was not a magician! Tell me what brings you to my abode?" The magician asked eagerly, his wise eyes glowing with curiosity and excitement as he placed a cup of tea in front of Elvis, and they both sat at a table in the house.

"I am on a journey to find the purpose of life," Elvis said quietly, before gulping down the hot tea that the magician had served him, it was delicious! Magical!

"Really," said the magician thoughtfully "that is a noble journey indeed. It is one I respect a lot. But tell me, as I am really curious, what have you found out so far?"

14

asked the magician picking up his own cup of tea and sipping from it.

"I have found that some people believe the purpose of life is to enjoy the earth, have fun in each moment and not worry about working hard, while others believe life's purpose is in staying away from the crowd and noise of others to find peace and truly enjoy life and nature and work hard to their satisfaction," said Elvis.

The magician smiled and said,

"Interesting"

"But you what do you believe is the purpose of life?" asked Elvis curiously.

"I believe in a combination of both actually, I believe the purpose of life is to live in the moment, enjoy each day, it's really not about working hard every time, but I also believe in working hard to use my magic to create buildings like this where I can have solitude, peace and work on whatever I want. I believe in enjoying each moment but also having the choice of solitude because I enjoy being able to stay alone without any crowd disturbing my concentration" answered the Magician with a wise twinkle in his eyes as he drank from his cup of tea again.

Elvis pondered his words feeling more confused than before, there were so many definitions of life, a lot of them intertwined and yet all so different.

So he stayed with the magician a few days before packing his bag and continuing on his journey after saying a hearty goodbye to him.

Elvis visited more people; the great cities of the wonderful inventors, the wealthy land of the businessmen, and even the Monks in their secluded towers of prayers.

They all gave him different answers and Elvis went back to his little house more confused than ever.

The Inventors taught him that the purpose of life was to create and make wonders with science.

The businessmen told him that the purpose of life was to work hard and make money.

"Life won't hand you anything, you have to take it!" They had said to him

The monks told him that the purpose of life was to live in peace with all men.

When he got home, Elvis found his grandmother waiting for him at the kitchen table, he told her all about his journey and explained all the confusing lessons he had learned on his way, so he asked her,

"Grandmother, what is the purpose of life?"

Grandma smiled and answered,

"To be happy and live life to the fullest by loving others with a heart free of burdens"

Elvis stared at her and wondered why everyone's answer was always so different, his grandma saw his confusion and decided to help.

"Elvis my dear the purpose of life might differ for each person but we all have one common ground; we all truly want to live. We want to know we achieved purpose and we want to experience life with a burning passion" she said smiling fondly at her grandson.

"Elvis the purpose of life for each person comes with pointers, they are the things that stir your heart and quicken your feet. They are the things you yearn for in the deepest recesses of your heart, they are special to you and your life's purpose does not have to be the same as anybody else's. It is yours, yours to fulfill, yours to live out. The path to purpose might come with hardships but never lacks pointers leading you to it. It might not make sense but taking each day one step at a time, you get closer to that purpose that makes your heart light up.

The only general thing is to share as much love as you can and live with a free, joyful, and kind heart. Laugh as much as you can, smile, forgive and share hope all around and life will begin to make sense and the path of purpose will become clearer" answered grandma.

Elvis stared at her in shock before giving her a big hug. The answer had been staring him right in the face all along!

So Elvis learned to enjoy each day and learn from each one, opening his heart, mind, and eyes to the pointers that were sure to come and each day began to make more sense and the purpose of life began to emerge.

THE SEARCH FOR ADVENTURE.

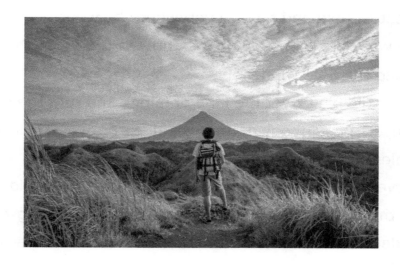

Once upon a time, the king of the wind lived in the far mountains up above, he was old and wise but couldn't move as fast as he could in his younger days, so he sent his sons; the three princes of the wind to blow through the earth, to cool down the land, to help nature in its course all over the world

They were the Northwind, the south wind, and the East wind. So the three princes of the wind blew; sometimes gentle, sometimes strong and sometimes like a great storm.

But one prince, in particular, turned out to be quite a trouble maker, blowing through the earth causing such great trouble and havoc everywhere he went.

He was the youngest of the three princes and he was called the East wind.

He would blow over the land of fairies and turn their little houses upside down, he would turn over their little tables, little chairs, and everything in sight. He would move with a great groan and scary sighs that would have all the fairies hiding under their beds and taking cover under the tables that he had turned over. The fairies were not a fan of the East wind and they wondered why he always caused so much havoc.

"It's the East wind again," The fairies said to one another, "he's quite a troublemaker" one fairy added, but still, they all hid under their beds and tables, scared of what more havoc the East wind was going to cause.

The East wind roared and screamed, scaring all the fairies, but he secretly laughed, enjoying all the chaos all around. When he was done there, he went on to the land of elves.

"I would be sure to have so much fun here," The East wind said to himself when he arrived in the land of the elves. He began causing chaos all over, with the elves scurrying to find a place to hide the minute they heard his scary roar and saw the wind carrying so much dust and chaos to them.

What a storm the East wind was brewing, turning everything in his path over and laughing when the elves screamed for help. He uprooted the plants, turned over the houses, and chased all the elves till they scurried into a sturdy hiding place.

What a day it was and oh how annoyed the elves were. They hid under the rocks and inside the caves, hearing the storm brewing outside, causing great chaos.

"The East wind is causing too much trouble, I do not like it," the leader of the elves said and the other elves nodded in agreement.

"We should report him to the king", said one little elf.

"Indeed we should" added the scared crowd of elves gathered in the caves.

"Yes, but first I shall report the East wind to his elder brothers, I'm sure they would talk some sense into him" answered the leader of the elves.

The elves were not happy with this decision as they listened to the great chaos the East wind was causing, they wanted to report him directly to the king but they knew how wise their leader was, so they agreed to report him to his brothers for now.

So together the fairies and the elves gathered to meet with the princes of the wind, and they did not go looking pleased in the least.

"Great princes of the wind, the ones we cannot see but can hear, the ones whose effect can be felt and can be seen, the ones who work with nature to help the earth, we greet you," said the leaders of the fairies and the elves.

"We greet you fairies and elves, the wonderful creatures who help mother nature and spread wonders all over the world. What brings you to our home in the mountains?" the two princes of the wind said, they were the South wind and the Northwind.

"We have come for a very serious reason oh princes. Why does your brother the East wind not act like you both? Rather he goes about causing havoc and destroying the hard work of the creatures, what wrong have we done to him? What does he aim to achieve by punishing us with so much chaos?" The leader of the fairies asked.

"Yes indeed, he blew so greatly all over our lands that we have been forced to rebuild and replant all over again. This is so much hard work and all the fairies and elves are angry, that is why we have come to make this known to you that you might speak to him to cease from causing such havoc" said the leaders of the elves

The princes of the wind were surprised to hear what their brother was doing and apologized to the fairies and the elves saying;
"We had no idea the East wind was doing anything like this, we are sorry and we apologize, we shall speak to him and ensure he behaves," said the brothers of the East wind.

"We understand and we look forward to your speaking to him", said the elves and fairies.

"Come eat and drink with us, before you return to your land, you have come a long way", said the Northwind, and all the fairies and elves were glad for the hospitality shown to them.
So they ate, drank and they rested, and when it was time to return home the Northwind and the south wind carried

them to their lands. The fairies and elves were very grateful and wondered how the two elder brothers were so kind and wise and the youngest was so unruly.

"I'm just glad we told them all about the unruly behavior of their brother and I'm sure they'll speak to him. If the East wind still doesn't listen then we shall report him to his father" said the leader of the fairies.

When the Northwind and the South wind called the East wind and asked him to explain the reason for his unruly behavior, he simply laughed about the dilemma of the elves and fairies.

"I am a prince of the wind, I go in search of adventure, I will not move at a slow pace like other creatures do, neither will I stay to the ground, because I am royalty. I am on the search for adventure, fun, and excitement, so I shall breeze through quickly, if it causes chaos so be it, I shall not live a boring life. I want to experience as much adventure and fun and when I speed through the land, I can feel the excitement burning in my body, I can't just settle for less and live like a tortoise. When I scale through the lands with a great sound and I cause the trees and houses to bow, I know I am having an adventure" said the East wind proudly.

"Oh East wind, you are getting it all wrong, the beauty of adventure is not in the speed, rather it is in the experience and that takes patience and understanding. Just speeding through houses, scaring creatures, and causing chaos isn't adventure, the real adventure is in the experiences you make along the way," answered the south wind.

"True adventure is in blowing gently, cooling the Earth and the people True adventure is in helping mother nature balance the air. True adventure is in seeing the smiles on the creatures' faces when they feel the gentle power of the wind as it cools, helps, and aids them through the day. True adventure is in traveling all over the earth as is your duty and learning from all the land, seeing the beauty they have, understanding their wisdom, and sending it all around. True adventure is in opening your eyes to the world around you as you travel East wind, not in causing chaos in the lives of the people" The North wind added.

The East wind pondered their words for a short while but soon he was prancing all over the earth causing chaos again.

This time he blew over the land of the humans, destroyed their houses, uprooted the plants, and made such great and scary sounds that the humans feared that the world was about to end.

Over and over he howled and everyone was sure the world would end.

The East wind enjoyed the chaos and soon he pranced to the animal kingdom and destroyed all he could find. What a mess he made!

He shook the mountains, he pulled out the trees and he blew over the oceans till they flooded the land. It was such a disaster!

This time all the humans, fairies, elves, and animals went straight to the King of the wind but they were greatly surprised when they got there to find the Northwind and the South wind already reporting the naughty East wind to their father. When the people saw this, they relaxed and listened to what the king of the wind had to say.

The King of the wind listened to his sons, and he was shocked at what he learned about his youngest son.

Then he listened to the elves and then the fairies and then the animals and then the humans and was even more dumbfounded by what they told him about the East wind.

The King listened to them and promised to settle it all.

"I greatly apologize for what my son has done and I promise that all your houses would be rebuilt and your trees would be replanted" answered the king. The people trusted him so they were appeased and knew that the wise king would do as he had promised.

That same day the king ordered the young prince to come back home.

The East wind was not remorseful when he arrived home, rather he pranced proudly in front of his father.

"Why did you do such a thing, my son? I am highly disappointed said the king.

"Father I am a prince, I need adventure, I cannot confine myself to following such rules and living a boring life," said the prince.

"Adventure is not chaos, rather it is experience. It is not in destruction but patience" the king said patiently but still, the East wind did not show any remorse.

"I see you have not learned a single thing, so this is what shall happen, you shall not be able to blow fast, or cause chaos. You shall be a gentle breeze, helping nature. You shall be forced to blow peacefully, cooling the land, helping the plants and you shall not have the speed to go fast" said the king, and immediately the prince lost all of his great speeding powers and could only blow like a gentle breeze.

"Noooo!!!' cried the prince at once.

Now the East wind is a gentle breeze, that cools you when you're hot, he's the teasing wind that blows gently through your hair and carries the relaxing sound of singing birds. The East wind is the gentle flow of air that chases heat out of a room. The East wind is learning what an adventure truly means, he's learning to patiently look at the earth as he travels, rather than speed through and leave chaos in his wake.

The East wind is experiencing the world, he no longer brings chaos and he's learning to be patient. The elves, fairies, animals, and humans love him. He doesn't rush through a land, rather he blows patiently, enjoying each moment, making friends with the people, understanding how they work, and helping the land to bloom and cool.

The East wind learned his lesson and when his father gave him back his powers, he never rushed through any moment again, he patiently helped, traveled, enjoyed the day and the night, traveled with eyes that could see and ears that could learn and he patiently experienced the adventures in every moment.

Together the three princes of the wind, blow through the earth and do wonders all around.

When you feel a cool, gentle breeze cooling you, teasing your hair, and bringing the sounds of birds to your ears, you know the prince of the East wind is nearby.

TOO MANY SPELLS ON TOO MANY DAYS

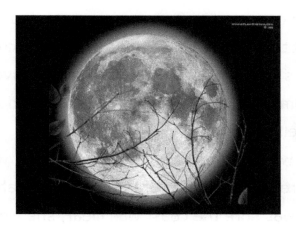

Once upon a time, there lived a fairy named Pat who was dreadfully lazy and loved to cheat every chance she got. If Pat needed anything, she would cast a spell to get it.

When Pat needed a cup of water, she was always too lazy to get up and would cast a spell for that too.
"Pat, it's wrong to use your powers like this. We fairies were not given powers to use selfishly or unreasonably. We are meant to use our powers to help nature and others. Why can't you get your cup of water yourself, why do you have to cast a spell for that too?" said Pat's mother, when she saw how increasingly lazy the young

fairy was becoming and how easily Pat abused her powers and cast spell for all the wrong reasons.

When Pat was told to do the dishes, she would look around, and to make sure no one was near then she would cast the spell of busy hands and all the cups, spoon and dishes would begin to wash themselves. When mother came back Pat would claim she had done all the work herself.
When pat was asked to clean the house, she would look around carefully to make sure no one was watching and when she was sure the coast was clear, she would cast a spell to make the house immediately clean without her having to do a single thing.

And when Pat was hungry, she would rather cast a spell to get some snacks rather than walk to the fridge to get them herself. Pat always looked for a way to avoid doing any work and abused her magic by casting spells for unrealistic things.

So, on and on the young fairy went, using magic to avoid doing any work.

When Pat spent her night going through the fairy magazine and tabs rather than going to bed, she would cast a spell the next morning so she wouldn't feel sleepy in the least.

Pat was always doing risky things with her magic and using her spells for things she should do herself.

"Pat why do you keep messing with magic and testing the limit of your powers by casting spells for silly things that you could do yourself. Magic isn't something to be tampered with or used carelessly" Mother always said but Pat never listened, she was always eager to find an easy way out using her magic.

Pat used her magic for incredibly simple things that she could do herself, like having her bath or brushing her teeth. She would stay up all night and wake up late the next morning, she would then be too tired to bathe or brush her teeth so she would cast the squeaky- clean spell so she would be clean without having to have her bath or brush her teeth.

One time the fairies had planned a picnic for all the young fairies and had asked if any fairies could help out with some snacks and baked condiments. Pat had proudly volunteered to help, despite knowing how lazy she was. She bragged and boasted of how much of a good baker she was. She pranced all over town telling everyone she would make the best cakes, pies, and scones ever for the picnic, but rather than settle down and learn to bake, Pat spent all her time lazing around, sleeping, and bragging. Then the day of the picnic came and Pat panicked, because she realized that all the other fairies would know how lazy she was.

Rather than plan or look for a way to bake the snacks, Lizzy spent all her time looking for a way to cheat and get the baked condiments without doing any work.
She spent hours looking through roll after roll of magic spell books, hoping to find a spell that would bake pies, scones, and cakes without her having to do any work.
So Pat spent a lot of time looking for a way to get the baked goods without actually baking anything. She searched and searched till she finally found the spell she needed.
She was really excited and cast the spell immediately and the baked goods appeared. She hurried off to the picnic and presented her baked goods to everyone and they all

oohed and ahead at the magnificence of what she had presented them.

Pat continued her bragging and boastful talks while everyone enjoyed the picnic.

When it was time to taste the baked goods, everyone was eager to eat Pat's snacks and when they did everyone soon realized Pat had cast a spell to bake the snacks because all the cakes, scones, and pies she had presented them tasted just like sand and it tasted horrible too.

The fairies were not pleased in the least and were very mad at Pat.

"If you couldn't bake the scones, pies, and cakes, Pat, you should have just told us! A lot of fairies were eager to help and bake for the picnic but you refused and now you've ruined the whole picnic! There's nothing anyone can eat here! How dreadful!" a fairy named Lizzy said, looking utterly annoyed.

The picnic was ruined and all the fairies were very sad and disappointed in Pat.

They couldn't eat a thing and simply sat, talked, and played and when they were all exhausted, they went back home, hungry and tired.

When they got back to the fairy village, they told everyone what Pat had done. Everyone was surprised that a fairy would use her magic for such simple tasks.

"Why did she offer to bake the cakes, scones, and pies, if she knew couldn't do them?" asked one of the adult fairies.

"I would never know why. She ruined the picnic, we had been planning it for over a year and Pat just had to ruin it, but you should have seen how she bragged, she bragged and bragged about being the best baker in all of fairyland only to mess up the whole day" Lizzy said sadly.

"It's okay Lizzy, fairies like her always get their reward in the end. Besides if this is how she misses her fairy magic for everything she needs to do, I'm sure she'll learn her lesson sooner rather than later" the adult fairy said.

Lizzy nodded sadly and went on her way.

When Pat's mother heard about what her daughter had done, she was greatly embarrassed and said to Pat;

"Pat, one must not misuse magic so, it leads to a lot of disaster in the end. We must learn to work hard because magic was not given to us so we could become lazy cheats, rather we have magic to help and beautify the earth"

"Oh, mother what is wrong with taking a few shortcuts in life. I didn't hurt anybody and nothing ever goes wrong when I use magic" Pat said confidently.
"I shall tell you a story and I hope it helps you see life in a different light." said her mother and so she began her story.

Once upon a time, there lived a very naughty fairy, who loved to cause a lot of trouble and cheat every chance he got

He would sneak to the village of the elves and steal all their fruits.
He would sneak into the magician's house and still his spell books too.
He was always causing trouble and never did a single chore.

He would lazy around all day using his magic to do everything, without getting up to work for a single moment.

The fairy was very lazy indeed.
Then one day, the little fairy needed to have his bath so he could go for a meeting of the fairies, which was happening in the skies, but just as was his usual ways, he was too lazy to get up and bathe himself.

All the other fairies had woken up early to go for the meeting, they had bathed, brushed their teeth, combed their air, worn clean clothes, and had flown to the sky for the meeting.
But since this fairy was so lazy, he simply lay in bed, twisting, turning, and yawning.
When he finally got up from his bed, he cast a spell to be squeaky-clean without having to bathe.

And the worst happened, the fairy turned into a statue, he turned into stone!
He couldn't open his mouth to call for help because he was now a statue and even if he could, there was no one

in the village to hear; every other fairy had gone for the meeting.

What a disaster it was.

The fairy was stuck for a long time before the other fairies finally came.

Even after that, no one knew he had turned to stone. It took a long time; close to 3years before anyone realized, and immediately they did, they cast a spell to free him.

The fairy was grateful but very exhausted, he immediately went to bed and slept for a long time and when he woke up, he promised never to be lazy or use his magic foolishly ever again.

Pat's mother said finishing her story.

After Pat heard the story, she was quiet for a while, but while her mother thought her daughter was learning the errors of her ways, Pat was simply thinking how foolish the lazy fairy had been to mess up his spells like that.

"I'm not that stupid, that could never happen to me," Pat said to herself.

"I've learned my lesson mother. I'll be more careful when it comes to using magic. I'll only use my magic for things

I need, not to lazy around" Pat said, smiling sweetly at her mother.

Her mother was so happy and hugged Pat proudly.

But Pat had not changed, she was only pretending.

So on the young fairy went, misusing her powers and causing havoc, the only difference was that now she was more careful and did not let anyone know that she was misusing her magic.

One day Pat's mother asked her to get some flowers from the garden. Now there is a strange relationship between fairies and flowers, and fairies are always warned to only cast spells on flowers that would help the flowers grow, blossom, and pollinate and that if they ever needed to cast a spell on a flower for any other reason, they needed to be very careful.

Pat remembered this but she was so lazy and said to herself
"I don't need to stress myself to pick the flowers. I'll just cast a spell" she said.

And so, she cast the spell and the flowers appeared in the house but when she tried to use her magic to bring a vase for the flowers, it didn't work.
She tried over and over again but it still didn't work!

Pat was alarmed and worried. She tried various spells but none of them worked! She had lost her powers! What a disaster it was.

She panicked and tried to find a solution; she picked up all the spell books she could find and tried all the spells in them that had anything on fairy powers, she mixed up strange plants that she hoped would help her get her powers back and she drank them, yet nothing worked.
Pat was near tears now and when her mother came back home, she tried to hide the fact that she had lost her powers.

But soon everyone in the fairy town came to know that Pat had lost her powers due to her lazy attitude. Everyone was shocked and amused as to how lazy a fairy could get to lose their power.
Pat had to learn to do all her chores from scratch and by herself, she had to learn to wake up early, have her bath,

sleep on time, brush her teeth, do the dishes and do all her chores by herself.

She had to learn to do everything without using her powers. And she enjoyed it! Pat had come to learn that there was a joy to life when we kept our hands and minds busy instead of looking for shortcuts

When all the fairies saw how hardworking she had become, they all decided to help her find a way to get her powers back.

They made concoctions after concoctions till they found the right one; the one that gave Pat the fairy her powers back.

Pat was elated when she got her powers back, so were the other fairies and Pat never cast a spell out of laziness again.

Rather she worked hard and only used a magic spell when it was very important or needed.

Her mind flourished and her hands became excellent at doing good, all because she decided to work hard rather than casting one too many spells.

THE QUEEN OF BELAM.

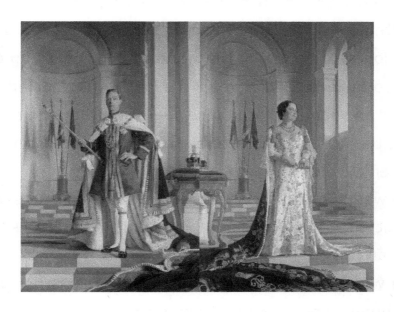

Once upon a time, there lived a beautiful princess who was wise, strong, and kind, she was the princess of the land of Belam. Her parents were very proud of her and they showed it by how they boasted of all her achievements and successes. They were eager to talk about all the good she was doing, they loved to listen to her, and they loved to sing her praises.

The princess was named Ruby and she was the apple of her parent's eyes.

As a little girl her father; the king loved to taker her with him to the royal library and show her all the many precious books it contained. He would read the books to her and watch as her eyes would glow in wonder and excitement as he read them to her. As she grew older, she loved to be lost in the world of books, curl up on a comfortable sofa and read the books till she left this world and floated through the pages, walking side by side with the fictional characters. Books were a blessing and she enjoyed every moment of them.

She would read on science; read about the planets, read about the atmosphere, read about the animals, the human body and so much more.

She would read about art; about the great artists, and the great works of art that had turned the world around, and about the various ways of creating wonderful works of art.

She would read about the business world; understanding the basic rudiments of every business, the wonderful history, and secrets of successful businesses, she would read and read till her eyes were heavy and her brain filled.

She loved the library, loved the books, loved the stories, and was overwhelmed by all the knowledge they held in their pages.

This wonderful princess loved to read till she was tired.

She was very knowledgeable and her parents were very proud of her. Whenever her father had a meeting with the council of elders, he would ask her opinion before every meeting as he prepared, because he knew she was very, knowledgeable, calm, and wise.

"What do you think of the issue that the council of elders is having a meeting on? The council of elders seems to believe that we should raise the taxes and focus on making the city more resourceful so more people can troop in and invest in the kingdom. What do you think of this?" Father asked her one morning as he ate breakfast, he was on his way to a meeting with the council of elders and he was having breakfast with his wife; the queen, and his daughter.

Ruby was quiet for a while as she pondered the question. "That seems like a very wise plan indeed father, but one has to realize that the people of the kingdom might not take this news happily, it should be expected that they might grumble, despite the fact that the decision is being made with their best interest at heart," Ruby answered as she buttered a slice of bread.

"I believe they should be eased into the idea and the details of the plans to make the kingdom more resourceful should be explained to them in detail. Their opinions should be taken into consideration and they should know they are an important part of this change. If you do things like this and ensure all the taxes are properly used, with the people in the kingdom being aware of how their taxes are being used, it will make the whole process seamless and beneficial with extraordinary results" Ruby said looking into the air thoughtfully
Her mother smiled proudly, giving the king a knowing look.
They both shared a smile and watched as Ruby returned to her breakfast.

"Very wise words indeed. Now tell me, my dear princess, would you like to accompany me to meet with the council of elders? " The king said and Ruby's slice of bread hung mid-air on its way to her mouth.

Ruby learned quickly and was a very valuable member of the council of elders and one could always see the king leaning to his right hand where she sat, to hear her opinion on every subject. She would whisper into his ears and he would give a satisfactory nod. Everyone knew that princess Ruby was wise and knowledgeable but her greatest strength lied in her kindness and her ability to see from the perspective of others.

Ruby was strong but yet gentle, she was opinionated and yet listened, she was disciplined and followed her schedule to the letter, yet she was kind and helpful to others who faulted.

The king could already see the makings of a great Queen in his child. He watched her proudly knowing his kingdom would end up in good hands with his daughter on the throne.

"Ruby, my precious jewel," said her mother one afternoon as they both sat in the garden, enjoying the warm sun and the gentle breeze.

"Yes, mother" Ruby answered in that gentle voice of hers.

"You have grown to be such a strong and wise woman and I am forever grateful that you are my child," The queen said

Ruby simply smiled "oh mother you shower me with so many compliments that I have to wonder how true each one is," she said

"Ruby there are no lies in my words, I have been blessed with a child who makes me happy indeed. What more could I ask for?" said the Queen.

"Besides now I know that when your father and I leave the throne you shall be able to take good care of the kingdom" the queen added.

Ruby shook her head with a gentle smile and said,

"You're going nowhere Mother"

Five years later; Ruby is a grown woman and has now been crowned Queen over the kingdom of Belam, the kingdom is flourishing and all the people love her.

Her parents had passed on and had left the throne for Ruby to fill.

She is young but wise beyond her years, beautiful and regal, yet kind and knowledgeable.

As the new queen reigned over the affairs of the kingdom, all can see great wonders and successes all around.

Changes in the kingdom, wealth all around.

The Queen was indeed wise and no one could say anything else. She listened patiently to every matter, she judged all the issues with wisdom and understanding. She took her time to make every decision, she was not one to make sudden verdicts and rules.

And so her kingdom flourished and the land bloomed.

But many rulers from other kingdoms did not believe she was wise or old enough to be king.

They considered her to be only a little girl and had severed business ties with her kingdom, yet it flourished and grew greater and greater.

Many Kings tried to sabotage all her decisions and plans but yet the young Queen found a way to always remain victorious.

There was one king in particular who was quite a trouble maker. He was the king of Westland.

He had a meeting with all the other Kings and Queens except Queen Ruby. He wanted to take over her kingdom because he considered her to be only a child.

"I welcome you all here again and I am very glad that you could all make it here." said the evil King
"Speak up, king of Westland, we respect you that is why we have come. Speak quickly as we all have a lot to do" said one king.

"Yes indeed, you are right, I shall go straight to the point. I want you all to work with me so we can wage war against the land of Belam and take it from the hands of the young Queen" the king of Westland said, and all the kings and Queens murmured among themselves, surprised by this decision.
At the end of the day, some of them agreed to work with him, while others refused, and yet there were others who were simply not interested.

Soon the plot began, first, they sent spies into the land of Belam, but the Queen was very wise and had been watching the stars at night through her telescope when the spies had entered the kingdom, she had ordered the guard to find them and bring them to the palace.

The spies were shocked that they had been discovered so quickly and feared for their lives. But rather than harm or punish them, she asked for them to be brought into the garden to meet with her, she spoke with them for a while but they refused to tell her who had sent them, or why.

The spies believed they would be killed eventually, so they decided to keep quiet. But the Queen surprised everyone yet again by her kindness, as she kept the spies in a house in the kingdom, and instructed guards to watch over the house, she fed the spies, clothed them, and was kind to them.

For several months the queen simply sent her good wishes, clothes, and food to the spies in their house.

The spies were confused at such kindness and eventually asked to see the Queen.

When they were brought to her presence, they bowed low saying, "the greatest Queen in all the earth, may you live long, longer than all who seek your ruin".

"Rise," said the queen as she wondered why they had asked to see her.

"We are very sorry that we came to your kingdom to do you harm, you have to realize that we simply did what we were asked," said the spies.

"It's fine, I understand. You see I mean no evil to you but I cannot let you go home and reveal whatever you have found out about my kingdom to whoever sent you if you refuse to tell me who sent you and why" said the Queen.

"We understand and that is why we have decided to help you. Other Kings and Queens, including the king who sent us, would have slain us without a moment's thought but you have been extremely understanding and patient so we must repay your kindness. It was the king of Westland who sent us, he together with some other Kings wish to take over your kingdom. We were sent to spy on your land and tell the king of Belam your weakness and the places where you were overtly confident" said the spies.

The Queen was not surprised, rather she nodded her understanding and asked what the spies would like to be done for them

"We would like to live in this kingdom as one of your people. We have seen the great wealth of your kingdom and would love to dwell in it. We have seen the love, patience, and kindness with which you rule your kingdom and we definitely want to enjoy it too. Grant us this one thing; that we dwell among your people as one of your own" answered the spies.

The Queen nodded her acceptance and asked that all they needed be provided for them.

And so the Kingdom of Belam grew in stature and might and more people came to dwell within its borders because of the great wisdom of the Queen that had caused great wealth.

When the king of Westland saw this, he was greatly vexed and roared in his kingdom like a wounded lion.

But he refused to give up, he sent more and more spies into the land but rather than return to him, they stayed in the land of Belam when they saw the great wealth and beauty of the land.

He didn't understand this and was confused. He invested and spent a lot of money in bringing down the Queen of Belam but all to no avail, nothing worked and the kingdom of Belam flourished.

He invested so much time in bringing down the Queen of Belam that he had not realized that his own kingdom was being destroyed by his own vengeance.

One morning he woke up and looked around his kingdom from a high point in his castle and he was immediately saddened by what he saw.

The land was desolate and barren, all the plants were dying and they looked poor and ugly. He had been so obsessed with bringing down the Queen that he did not realize that he had been destroying his own kingdom.

After many days he sneaked into Belam himself and what he saw shocked him.

The land was beautiful, amazing and a wonder to behold.

The streets were lined with gold and all the citizens looked wealthy, wealthier than the king himself!

He sneaked to the castle and saw all the other Kings and Queens dining with the Queen of Belam.

The same Kings and Queens who he had convinced to stand against her, somehow, they were now working with her, instead of him.

He marveled at the great wisdom of such a young Queen and sadly returned to his kingdom.

He promised to change his ways and began to work hard to be a good and wise king, rather than an evil one.

And slowly his land flourished and his kingdom grew, he never again stood against the Kingdom of Belam, he sang the praises of the young Queen and talked all about her wisdom.

CHRISTMAS WITH LANA

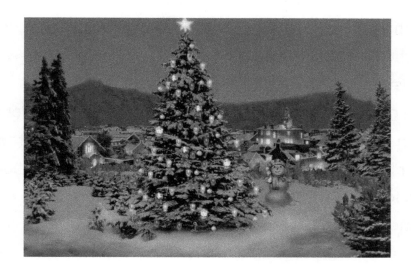

Lana stared out the window and watched as the snow fell, slowly, steadily, adding to the already festive air all around. She hugged herself tighter in the sweater which she wore and drank hot coffee from the mug in her hands. A sad sigh escaped her lips as she lowered the mug from her lips and stared out the window and watched the snowfall, she hated the holidays.

From where she sat at her window, she could see families walking happily, hand in hand, Christmas shopping bags in hand, and looking elated as they enjoyed the festive atmosphere.

She heard the laughter of children, she saw the smiles on the faces of couples as they walked hand in hand, love in their eyes as they enjoyed the joy that came with Christmas. A joy that came to others except her.

She grimaced, stamped her feet on the floor, and got up from her cozy sit by the window. Having to watch these people and realize they had a wonderful life and probably had lots of warmth and excitement waiting for them back home was always a pain for Lana to watch.

She headed to her bedroom and jumped underneath the sheets, eager to close her eyes and lock away the smiles, the laughter, the joy, and the love she had seen in the eyes of all the people she had watched from her apartment window. The holidays were a constant reminder of all she never had. The holidays were a reminder of all she lost. It felt like the world held a banner high above its head aimed at reminding her that her life was a boring, lonely facade.

She rolled her eyes from underneath the sheets. She just had to survive another holiday season, just like she did every other year. All she had to do was survive…

She woke up to the constant ringing sound of a phone beside her.

She grumbled from her sleep and sleepily swiped at the noisy monster that was disturbing her night rest. She mumbled to herself and dozed off again when the horrible ringing stopped but just when the room had fallen totally silent and Lana had dozed off to the land of dreams, the phone began ringing again, seemingly louder than before and with a vengeance to wake up any being in its path.

This time Lana sat up on her bed with a huff, looking around angrily to find the ringing monster that had ruined her sleep.

Her eyes still dim with sleep made out her cellphone laying on the bedside table and she groaned and reached out, grabbing it.

"Hello," she said into the phone sleepily

"Hey you" the voice from the other end answered

She pulled the phone away from her ear to take a look at the collar I.D.

It didn't show any name.

"Mikey, did you change your phone number?" she said into the phone as she got up heading to the kitchen to make herself some coffee so she could actually wake up. Her mind was still in a sleepy haze and she kept tripping and knocking into things on her way to the kitchen, she really needed that coffee.

"Naa, I'm at a friend's place my phone is dead so I decided to use hers," Mikey said into the phone, and Lana's eyes immediately lit up and her lips curled into an excited smile.
Mikey had been her best friend from kindergarten, all the way to adulthood. He was more of a brother now, and people actually considered them to be siblings not that she could blame them, they were both curly-haired brunettes, who were always together but that was as similar as they got, while Mike was tall and muscular, Lana was petite.

While Mike was outgoing and gentle, Lana was a fire-breather but also a loner. They weren't similar in the least but somehow, they had remained best of friends all these years. I guess opposites did attract.

"You're with her!" Lana said with so much excitement in her voice.

Mikey gave a throaty laugh "Yes..." he whispered into the phone.

Lana felt like jumping, Mikey was at Stacey's, she was a girl Mikey had been hitting on for the past year and he had not gotten around to telling her how he felt or even hanging out with her. If he had slept over at her place that was a good thing, a wonderful thing!

"You slept over?" She asked barely able to hold back her excitement

Mikey gave a nervous laugh "yes..."
This time she did a little victory dance in her room-
"We're staying over at her parents for Christmas" she heard Mikey say and Lana paused in confusion.
"Uhn?"

"I'm sorry Lana, I know we always spend Christmas together, but Stacey invited me over to have Christmas with her and her parents and I couldn't say no," Mikey said apologetically and Lana froze.
She had no one, no one except Mikey. This Christmas was going to be the worst one yet.

"Lana? Lana?" Mikey said into the phone

"Why?" She heard herself say softly

"I'm sorry, I'll explain everything when I get back okay...
I'm sorry... Lana..."

"You know I have no one, absolutely no one!" She yelled
into the phone
"And I'm sorry, just...call Suzy, I'm sure she'll have
something planned out for Christmas," he said and she
heard the hope in his voice, she sniffed, so he really was
that eager to get rid of her.

"I haven't talked to her in weeks and besides Suzy
doesn't check up on me, I'm not going to hit her up now
like some needy cheapskate"

"Uhmmm...okay you could call Nelson, he'll love to hang
out," Mikey said hopefully

"No, he missed my birthday and barely calls me," she
said sighing as she relaxed against the kitchen counter

"But he's your friend..." Mike said

"Well, now he's only your friend. He's just an acquaintance to me now" she said picking out imaginary dirt from her fingers.
She heard Mikey sigh and she knew he would be dragging a hand down his hair

"Give Maggy a call?" He asked
"No, she's always flaunting her baby and marriage in my face like it's some type of-"

Mikey cut her short" stop Lana, just stop okay...can't you see... you're- you're bitter and hateful and judgemental. Why don't you give people a chance I promise you it's a whole lot better to live life that way... Lana, you're my best friend and I love you. Can't you see that's why no one hangs out with you anymore, it's because you're always nagging, complaining, and being a general pessimist"

"Wow," Lana said and she hated the way her voice cracked.

"I'm sorry but I just want the best for you and living life so lonely and-"

"It's fine Mikey, now I know why we're not spending time together. I'm bitter, hateful, judgemental, and lonely" She said into the phone feeling dejected.

"Lana no... I love you; you know that- I mean you know that right? I want you to be happy, reach out to any of our friends, I'm sure they'll be glad to have you over. You don't have to wait for them to reach out first, uhn?" He asked and his voice had that calm, concerned and caring tone that normally would have soothed her but right now just irked her.

So she remained silent.

"Lana?" She heard him say from the other end but she simply remained silent.
"Lana I -" Mikey was saying but a woman's voice interrupted him. It had to be Stacey.
Mikey

She heard the voice say and Lana bristled, she had been the only one to call him Mikey since they were kids. Stacey was suddenly a pain.

"Lana, I have to go, call me okay?" He said into the phone urgently

"Lana, I just want the best for you, loads of love and Merry Christmas," he said with a resigned tone before hanging up the call when she didn't reply.

She stared at the phone for the longest time before walking slowly back to bed. Christmas was ruined and there was no helping it.

It had been hours since she had been up and she had been staring at the phone with a mixture of both anger and hope

Maybe Mikey was right.

She was always angry over every detail that went wrong with a friend, if someone didn't call her first, she immediately held a grudge.

She was quick to cut off friendships,

She never reached out first,

And she constantly highlighted all the wrongs in others.

She sighed as she stared at the tiny booklet in her hands.

Was Mikey, right?

"I can't reach out first because I'm always so busy," she said out loud to herself
Well, what if they're busy too, Her mind said and she immediately sobered up

She thought for a while then she said out loud again " well I want to call sometimes but I don't want to be a bug or inconvenience, anyone"

"What if that's how they feel too, we all need someone to reach out to us, we all need company and it doesn't matter who reaches out first, the point is to reach out and be there for one another," her mind said and this time she laughed because she knew that was what Mike would have said, but it was a sad laugh, knowing she wouldn't be spending Christmas with her best friend.

She sighed, took one last long look at that booklet that had tons of phone numbers that she had deleted from her mobile out of anger and hurt.
First, she called Maggy.

"Lana?" The voice at the other end sounded both surprised and cautious.
"Yes..." Lana said skeptically, she was ready to end the call and high tail it out of there.

"Hi... how - how have you been? I missed you, you know "Maggy said sadly and all of Lana's fear evaporated. She had been living in her mind, everyone wanted company.

Soon they talked, and talked, and talked, catching up on every detail. And Lana bagged herself an invite to a Christmas party

With that confidence, she called friend after friend.
Laughing, smiling, crying, rebuilding past relationships was wonderful.

Even Nelson sounded so happy to hear from her, he had had a rough year and had said her voice was like a soothing balm in these tough times. He was coming over to hang out tomorrow. Lana was elated.

She was actually going to organize a Christmas Eve party at her house because so many of her friends were coming over. She gave a sad laugh, we were all similar, weirdly, no one wanted to be an island forever and loneliness was no one's dream, reaching out did wonders to the heart.

By the time she curled up for bed that night, she was smiling so much that it hurt, and her phone was still receiving texts from friends who were so eager to catch up.

She found herself laughing as she read each message, she had been a fool to isolate herself in such bitterness and loneliness, now if only Mikey could be here.

Maybe she would tell him she loved him and not as a friend but as much more, way much more.

The thought dampened her mood, she shook her head and gave a lazy smile, Mikey was her best friend and he and Suzy were having a wonderful Christmas, he deserved all the good he could get.

She woke up slowly, it was Christmas Eve!

She jumped up, pulled back the curtains, and opened the windows,

"Merry Christmas!" She yelled to everyone on the streets.

They looked up in confusion but soon everyone was waving and yelling "Merry Christmas!" back at her. She smiled, reaching out first wasn't so bad after all.

She brushed her teeth, freshened up, and was preparing for her party when her phone rang.

"Hey, Nelson!" She said happily

"Hey Lana, what do you think I should get for the party, I'm packing up my bag and I just need to know how much space I have left," Nelson said laughing, Lana giggled.

"Just bring yourself Nel, come quick, I'm not about to set up for a party all by myself," she said as she tried to decide what type of wine to bring upstairs from the cellar

"I'll hurry, bye"

"Bye"

She dropped the phone with a smile and the doorbell rang just as she got to the kitchen.

She stared at the clock, that was fast of Nelson.

She hurried to the door

"Nelson, how in the world-" her eyes went wide and she stopped mid-sentence when she saw who was at the door.

"Merry Christmas Lana" Mikey said with his boyish smile, looking apologetic and her knees turned to butter.

But instead, she frowned, left the door open, and stalked inside.

He followed after her silently

"Merry Christmas," he said and he walked by her to place a box in the center table.

He looked around the house, obviously surprised at the party decorations all around

She shrugged, embarrassed, and said "I guess I'm having a party"

He gave a throaty laugh, the kind that always had her senses in a mess. That was the last thought passing through her mind before he leaned down and placed a kiss on her lips.

Her brain froze and her lips responded of their own accord.

Mikey lifted his head and traced his hands across her lips. "I'm sorry about what I said, I love you Lana and when I say I love you I mean it is as way more than a friend, and it's fine that you don't feel the same way I just want you to-" she was the one who interrupted him by pulling him in for another kiss and soon they were both cuddled together on the sofa wondering how they had both missed that they had feelings for each other that went beyond friendship all these days.

"What about Stacey?" Lana asked in confusion

"She needed my help to set up for Christmas and I finished earlier than I thought," he said staring at her like she was the most important person in the world.
"But I thought-"
"You thought I liked her, didn't you?" Mikey asked.
"Well yes," she said sitting up

Mikey laughed " I picked a random name to tell you how much I liked you, thinking somehow you would get the hint but as unlucky as I am, you hunted down a Stacey, and it turned out I did have a Stacey at work. I couldn't tell you the truth that all the feelings I had been describing were feelings I had for you and that I had never even known that there was a Stacey at my office till you forced me to say hello to her" Mikey said scratching his neck with an embarrassed laugh

"But I told her you liked her" Lana said looking confused.

"Yeah... she knew that was a lie so I told her the truth from the start, she knew you were the one I was in love with, "Mike said placing a gentle kiss on her forehead

Lana gave a shocked laugh.

"Mikey..."

"Merry Christmas Lana"

******.

It was the most amazing party ever; all her friends were together and the excitement was off the charts

"So, you sneaky little monsters!!" Nelson said to her and Mike over the music, as they all sat together laughing and enjoying the food and the joy of Christmas.

Lana rolled her eyes and Suzy gave her a tight hug " I missed you" she said leaning in and resting her head on Lana's shoulder.

The house was filled to the brim with friends from all over and Lana had never felt happier, reaching out first wasn't so bad after all. It just showed we were all human, and we needed each other and Lana was glad Mikey had taught her that.

THE BAKER

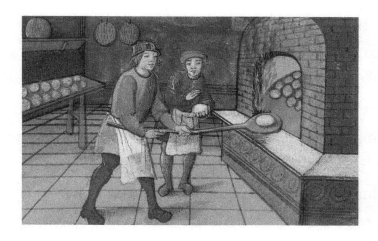

Once upon a time, there lived a baker, who baked the most amazing bread in all of the kingdom of Memphis. He would roll, knead and then bake the bread in the ovens at extremely high temperatures, one could perceive the aroma from all over town, it always smelled wonderful and mouthwatering no matter the time of day. From far and wide people would keep popping into the bakery to buy the wonderful bread. The bread smelled wonderful and it tasted ten times better too.

The bakery was always so warm and welcoming, the bread so hot and soft that it melted in your mouth once it touched your tongue.

It was a wonderful place to come to, it was a wonderful place to eat.

The baker was friendly and eagerly welcomed all the customers that came from far and wide to taste his floured goodness. He ensured all his bread were baked to perfection and all over Memphis no baker could compare to this great baker, but most of all the baker was so kind and gentle that many claimed it was his kindness that made him such a great baker.

When you asked him what his secret to such amazing baked wonders, he would laugh and continue kneading the dough.

Far and wide fairies, elves, wizards, sorcerers, sorceress', dwarves and so many other mystical creatures came to the bakery to buy bread from the baker. No one ever had a single complaint and more people kept coming from far and wide to buy his hot and tasty bread. Kings and Queens promised him great rewards if he would only come to their palace and be their baker, but the baker kindly refused and always returned to his bakery.

One time the king of a far land heard about his baked goodness and sent a letter requesting him to come to his palace and work as the royal baker, but the baker again kindly refused and remained in the city of Memphis baking for all who came from far and wide to buy his bread.

The king from this far land was not pleased and asked all the bakers all over his kingdom to bring their bread to him to taste so he could prove to the baker from Memphis that he had bakers that were even better than him in his kingdom.

So, all the bakers in this far land brought their bread to the king excitedly, but the more he tasted, the more he realized there was no baker in his kingdom as good as the baker from Memphis.

He was greatly angered and wrote a very stern letter to the baker at Memphis asking him to come at once!
He then turned to the bakers in his Kingdom
"So, does it mean not even one of you can make bread like the baker of Memphis! How shocking, that you do not know such quality" the king said, shaking his head in disappointment.

"How can you call yourselves royal bakers and you can't make bread that melts in the mouth, full of so much buttery goodness, so hot that it warms your soul, gentle on the tongue and yet does wonders to the taste buds" added the king, with a wistful light in his eyes.

The baker from Memphis replied to the king from the far land again, kindly refusing, eventually the king came to Memphis himself to visit the baker and he ate as much bread as he could ever want.

Tasty, soft, buttery, milky bread, so delicious, so mouth-watering, so enticing, that the king ate and ate, till he could eat no more.

He was greatly pleased and said to the baker.

"You have done well; you are indeed the greatest baker ever. If you do ever change your mind, know there is a place for you in my royal palace. Now I best be on my way, thank you for the delightful loaves of bread. Have a good day my friend" the king said happily, patting the baker on his back. Before the king left, he gave the baker a big bag of gold and lots of precious gifts that shocked all around, especially the baker himself.

When some of the bakers from the far land heard this, they were greatly angered and wanted to find out the secret of the great baker from Memphis. So, they came to Memphis and pretended to be curious tourists who wanted to have a taste of the bread and know all about how it was made.

The baker was elated
"Come, come in, see the inner kitchen where the kneading and baking take place," the baker said eagerly when they told him they wanted to know how he made such wonderful bread.
The bakers from the far land were surprised by his hospitality, kindness, and generosity. They wondered why he eagerly showed them his kitchen and explained the baking process to them.

They were very glad that now they knew his secret and would be able to bake just as well as he did and even better.

So, they thanked the baker still pretending to be curious tourists and hurried back to the far land.

They were very eager to try out the baker's procedure in their own bakeries and immediately they got home they set to work, testing, kneading, and baking the cake just like they had seen the baker at Memphis do.

They made bread and immediately took it to the king to have a taste feeling satisfied and proud of what they had made.

The king was just as excited, asking for the best plates, spoons, and cups to be presented to him as he dined on the wonderful bread that the bakers had made.
But the minute he took the first bite, his face paled and he spit out the bread. It tasted horrible!
He stared at the bakers in shock
"What is this! What are you trying to do! Even the cattle in my backyard can bake something better than this! Take this horrendous mess away from me!", The king barked in anger.

The bakers were embarrassed beyond comprehension and shamefully took their bread back to their bakeries.
 When they got there, they tasted the bread and even they were overwhelmed by how horribly it tasted.

"That baker from Memphis must have deceived us!" yelled one of the bakers

"But we watched him mix the dough, he did it right in front of us and we tasted it once it was baked," said another baker

"Yes indeed, but he might have switched the mixture when we weren't looking or... how else do you explain this horribly tasting bread?" Asked one of the bakers.

"Indeed, you are right. He played a fast one on us!" answered another.

The bakers were greatly annoyed and looked for a way to get back at the baker of Memphis since they believed he had taught them a wrong recipe on purpose. So, they plotted and planned.

"We shall have to look for a way to get back at him. We'll see how funny it looks when he's the one being embarrassed in front of his customers." The bakers said, laughing with evil glee.

After a few days, they decided on a plot that would definitely ruin things for the baker at Memphis just as he had ruined things for them as royal bread makers.

They visited a wizard in their city.

"This is a lotus flower, once you place it in the dough it will be ruined and will taste horrible. It also has magical powers that will make sure no one comes back to by bread from this baker once they smell the lotus flower in the bread," said the wizard.

The bakers were glad and immediately set on a journey to Memphis so they could get revenge on the baker.

The baker at Memphis was glad to see them and asked how they were.

He invited them into his bakery again and even served them lots of delicious bread for free.

The bakers enjoyed the bread but still, they planned to ruin it with the lotus flower.

When the baker walked out to speak to a customer, they sneaked into the kitchen and sprinkled the lotus flower all over the dough, and kneaded it into it. When they were satisfied with the amount of lotus flower they had added, they quietly returned to their sits, eager to watch the disaster that was sure to come.

The baker returned into the kitchen unsuspecting and put the dough in the oven. When the bread was ready, he served it to his customers, the evil bakers laughed with glee, glad that their plan was working.

But to that surprise, rather than for people to be disgusted and hate the bread, they ordered for more and more and more!

The bakers stared in confusion as all the bread in the bakery ran out.

They stared at one another in surprise but still, they refused to give up.

Soon when the baker stepped out again, they sneaked into the inner kitchen and added more lotus flower to the dough, again the baker walked in unsuspecting and put the dough in the oven.

And this time when the bread was ready, a throng of people pushed into the bakery, each all-throwing money at the baker, eager to get a piece of his bread. The evil bakers stared at one another in confusion, the lotus flower was making people rush for the bread rather than make them be disgusted by it.

They stared in shock and confusion as all the bread ran out again. This time they did not bother to try to add any more lotus flower to the dough, rather they ran out and ran all the way to their kingdom, confused by the happening at Memphis.

When they got their own bakery, they decided to try the lotus flower on the bread.

"Maybe the wizard was wrong and the lotus flower actually works for good rather than bad," said one of the evil bakers.
"Indeed, can you see how the baker at Memphis' bakery improves the more we put the lotus flower in the dough? I bet if we put it in our dough, the king and everyone else in this kingdom would fall in love with our baking" said another baker.
All the bakers nodded in agreement and gladly added the lotus flower to their baking, then they shared the bread all over town but to their surprise everyone hated it!

Even the king! And no one wanted to taste bread made by them ever again. The king even ordered that their title as royal bakers be revoked!

The bakers could only stare in confusion and fear, wondering what was going on.

They hurried to visit the wizard and asked him what had gone wrong.

"We live in a strange world, that baker from Memphis did not lie to you, he showed you exactly how he baked his bread. You see his bread tasted so good because he has done good to a lot of people and they are constantly wishing him well and praying for his success. It is their good wishes that make whatever he bakes so perfect. You, on the other hand, have offended quite a lot and have lived a selfish and self-centered life and that is why your bread does not taste as wonderful as his does. The lotus flower is magical and it respects a man that carries a lot of good wishes like that baker and that is why the lotus flower did the opposite of what it was meant to do and made more people demand the bread." Answered the wizard.

The bakers were shocked and walked back to their homes slowly.

They decided to be kinder, share, and be less vengeful from that day on and things began to change.

More people enjoyed their bread and even the king called them back to service in the royal kitchen.

Rather than try to pull others down, they encouraged and helped them and they flourished.

And they learned that the first secret to being a good baker was a good heart because that was where everything all started.

ELEANOR AND THE SHIP

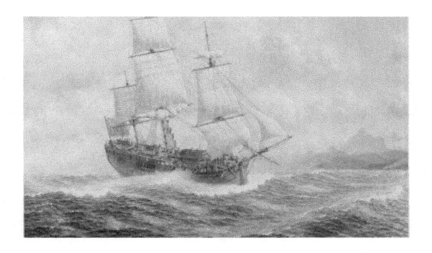

Ella was always so curious and dreadfully restless. She was up before the early hours of dawn, peeping through her window, wondering if adventure would come to her today. During breakfast as she ate in the cozy kitchen with her mother and father, she would stretch so she could look out the window and try to see if anything interesting was outside.

Before lunch she would stand outside the door, peering, searching in the bushes, picking up shiny stones and metals, and then run around the yard in one last attempt to find adventure.

And when it was time for dinner her eyes would be heavy, her body exhausted, and her mood down because she didn't find any adventure today.

The next morning, she would wake up in the early hours of the morning, unable to get enough sleep, and then she would repeat the process all over again; the search for adventure.

Today she peered out the window, expecting the same boring routine of finding nothing, but surprisingly this time there was something very, very interesting on the lake just behind her house. She rubbed her eyes, to make sure she wasn't hallucinating.

There really was a ship on the lake! And it was massive too! Ella ran down the stairs in excitement, rushed through the sitting room, and was just about to open the back door in the kitchen and head to the lake when mother called her.

"Eleanor Mary Roosevelt!" Mother called and Ella cringed.

When mother called her name in full, especially with her middle name, Ella knew there was trouble in sight.

"Yes, mother," Ella said putting on her brightest smile.

"Where do you think you're going?" Mother asked, standing with her hands on her hips and looking stern.

"Ummm...to the...you see there's a ship...you see and I just... I just need to take a glimpse, nothing much just a glimpse and I'll be right back" Ella said smiling brightly and rocking on the balls of her feet, with her hand folded in front of her.

"Take a look at yourself," mother said and she did not look amused.

Ella slowly looked down at her clothes, she was still wearing her nightgown, she was also barefooted and when she slipped a hand through her hair, she realized it was a mess, like a raven's nest.

Ella grimaced and bowed her head.

"And I believe I don't need a soothsayer, to say exactly how your room looks, do I?" Mother asked and this time she had an amused smile on her lips.

Ella did not even wait to give a reply, rather she hurried up the stairs and all the way to her room.

When she got to her room, she collapsed on her bed with a sigh and groan, then she remembered the ship and she jumped up and headed to her window so she could get a better look. It was beautiful and it glowed in the early morning sun as the sun rays bounced off its body.

Ella's smile returned in full force and she hurried to clean up her room.

She arranged her bed, made sure the sheets were straightened out, and placed the pillows properly.

Next, she looked at the walls in her room that were painted a bright purple and she adjusted all the picture frames on them and Eleanor had quite a number of picture frames on these walls. She was proud of every single picture and she adjusted them carefully.

Next, she grabbed a broom and began to sweep the floor of her room but the dust that rose from it was tremendous. Eleanor ran out in shock at how dusty her room floor was.

Her mother came to stand beside her just outside the room and they both watched her bedroom as it was covered in a cloud of dust.

"Yes... I know, it's a disaster...now get to work Eleanor"
Mother said and she continued walking down the corridor
and then she took the stairs and Eleanor watched her
decent.

She turned her eyes slowly to see the dusty room again
and she cringed at the mess in front of her.

How was she ever going to finish this if she was going to
get to the ship?

She stretched and stood on tiptoes so she could see the
lake from above the clouds of dust in her room.

It was still there!

She looked at the broom with determination glinting in
her eyes and she set to work.

Next, she hurried, and found a mop and bucket and
cleaned the floor.

She got a stool and cleaned all the windows, then she
fixed up her closet and her reading table which was at
the far end of the room just by the second window in her
room.

For the next few hours Eleanor simply cleaned and
cleaned till her room sparkled and smelled like roses, she

stepped into the bathroom and washed it till she could see her reflection in the now shiny tiles.

She gave a smile of satisfaction, and watched the beautiful room, beholding all the hard work she had put in today. Never had she worked so hard.

She looked at the window and blew a kiss at the ship by the lake.

"Hold on my hope for adventure, I'm coming for you," Eleanor said gladly and she hurried to clear out all the cleaning supplies and have her bath.

*****

The only sounds in the room were the ticking of the clock and the silent rhythm of Eleanor's breath as she slept.

The adventurous hard worker was utterly exhausted from all the hard work she had put in today and was sleeping soundly.

Her breath formed a timeless rhythm with the sound of the clock. The clean and quiet room felt, looked, and smelt like a haven.

The bed looked crispy clean, the floors glittered and one could see their reflection on them, the windows were bright and clean and the moon shined brightly into the room. One could make out the ship on the lake.

The reading table by the second window was neatly arranged with roses in a vase, placed daintily on it. The room held the wonderful scent of the roses.

And Ella slept soundly like one who didn't have any worries at all.

*****

The next morning Ella woke up utterly astounded, how had she forgotten about the ship! She stared in confusion, at the bed and her room.

She must have slept off after cleaning the room but how come no one woke her up.

She stretched and yawned as she stood up from her bed and headed straight to the bathroom. She stumbled a little and squeezed her eyes open and close again to take the sleep and tiredness away.

She was really stiff, how long had she slept.

She checked the wall clock just by the toilet door.

It was 7 am!

She had slept for 14 hours?

Ella shook her head, wow, she must have been more exhausted than she had thought. She squinted against the sunlight and saw the Ship, excitement pulsed in her veins and she hurried to have her bath.

She made sure her room was clean and then she dressed up and headed down the stairs. When Ella got downstairs, she checked the mirror in the hallway before stepping into the sitting room to say hello to her mother and father.

"Hello-", the words froze on her lips, her parents were having breakfast with sailors and what looked like a ship captain, Ella eyes widened, could it be? It had to be? The ship on the lake?

Ella looked at the kitchen door before turning o look at the sailors in her house. Real life sailors in her house.

Mother turned just in time to see her.

"Ella you're up, finally you woke up, you've been asleep for hours" mother said with an endearing smile and Eleanor walked over to give her a hug and a kiss on the cheek and she did the same for father as was their morning greeting.

"Captain Jack, meet my daughter Eleanor Mary Roosevelt," her father said beaming proudly. Ella was just glad she had brushed her teeth, had her bath, combed her hair, and worn clean clothes before coming downstairs.

"Hello Eleanor, it's nice to meet you," the captain said smiling brightly, he had kind green eyes that had Eleanor smiling back at him.

"You can call me Ella, everybody does," Ella said, still smiling.

"Why of course, these are two of my crewmen, Micheal and Taylor and this is my son Jackson junior and my daughter Drusella," said the captain proudly.

It was then Ella noticed a boy and girl who were just about her age seated at the far end of the sitting room, watching the television, she had not been able to see them earlier because she had been so focused on the sailors.

Ella hurried over to say hello, it had been a while since she had seen children her age come to visit, so seeing these two children made her very glad.

"Hello, nice to meet you," she said as she joined them on the settee to watch the television with them.

The girl named Drusilla smiled brightly "nice to meet you too. I'm so glad I got to meet a child my age" Drusella said and before Ella could reply Jackson Junior interrupted saying,

"Yesterday we came to play but your mother said you were asleep. Do you always sleep for so long?"

Ella laughed, shaking her head "No I cleaned my room for so long that I was so exhausted and just fell asleep once I was done" she said

"It must have really been messy," Jackson said smiling, he had green eyes just like his father, and they glowed with friendliness and joy.

Ella liked them both already. Drusella's eyes were more emerald than green and they glowed with such a lovely intensity that you wanted to look at them all day, she had fiery red hair and a gentle smile that looked angelic, Ella couldn't help but smile back at the angelic beauty.

"Would you like to show us your room?" Drusella asked with her eyes wide.

Ella nodded eagerly, she had cleaned this room for hours, she would gladly show it off.

So together all the children raced up the stairs and Ella proudly presented her room to them.

"Wow," said Drusella "it's so neat and pretty" she added.

Ella smiled

"It's bright and colorful," Jackson said and Ella beamed.
"Would you like to see our room on the ship? It's decorated just like our room back home" Drusella said smiling.
And Ella's heart skipped a beat, an opportunity to get to touch, walk, and see that beautiful ship up close? Ella wouldn't reject it for the world!

She raced ahead of the children, all the way out of the house and headed straight for the lake.
She heard their giggling behind her as they hurried to catch up with her.
When Ella finally made it to the lake, she could only stare in awe. The ship was a beauty, a dream, standing with such magnificence and splendor under the glowing sunlight.

"It's beautiful isn't it?" Jackson whispered beside her, and Ella could only nod.
"Come on, let's go in," Drusella said

Ella couldn't believe she would actually get to enter the ship.

Together the children walked into the ship and the crew members working on the ship said hello to drusella and Jackson, and the children introduced Ella to all of them and then they said hello to her also.

The crew was very friendly and happy as they worked together. Finally, the children got to Drusella's room, it was fit for a princess, and it was clean too! Eleanor's eyes widened,

"Wow," she said.

"Come let me show you my room," said Jackson, pulling Ella with him and when she walked into his room, she wasn't any less stunned.

Ella felt so proud to be able to stand among these two children with clean beautiful rooms on a ship, knowing she had a clean and absolutely beautiful bedroom too.

She smiled happily; the ship was amazing!

But slowly the image of the children, the ship, and the rooms began to disappear and Eleanor woke up on her bed and she stared in confusion at the place around her.

She was meant to be on a ship!

She stared out the window, the ship stood regal and beautiful under the sun.

She looked at her room, clean and sparkling, then why was she not on the ship?

She had her bath, cleaned her room, dressed up, and hurried down the stairs.

When she got to the sitting room, she met her parents having breakfast with some sailors just like in her dream and captain Jack who she had seen in her dream! She stretched and saw two children; a boy and a girl watching television at the far end of the sitting room, it was Drusella and Jackson!
Mother turned just in time to see her and spoke "Ella you're up, finally you woke up, you've been asleep for hours," mother said with an endearing smile and Eleanor walked over to give her a hug and a kiss on the cheek and she did the same for father as was their morning greeting, but this time she did it with a broad smile on her lips.

She had dreamt about today!
And she couldn't wait for the adventure to begin.

ANNE AND THE ELVES

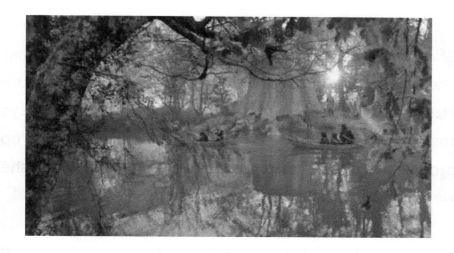

All the children of the Elvis family had to do a chore, each morning they would all go about their duties like skilled workers, with all their attention focused on finishing their duties so they could go out and play.

Anne was the youngest of the five children in the Elvis family, she was also the most curious of all five I, she was constantly asking questions about everything, observing things that no one else did, and having answers for the most hidden mysteries.

She had a smile that was as bright as the sun and eyes that glowed with curiosity, knowledge and a love for life that had everyone who walked by her to keep turning back.

She had wavy dark brown hair that stopped at her shoulders and mother said it gave her the look of a cute little pixie, when mother said that, a happy giggle always rose from Anne's insides and she would hold her head up proudly when she went about her chores or when she went to play with the other children.

Anne was just 13 years old but she was sharp, witty, and as curious as a cat. She loved to play outdoors so it was no surprise that she got the chore of heading to the grocery shop to get the bags of flours needed each day.

Mrs.Elvis; Anne's mother, had a bakery and all the children helped out at the bakery, and it was the most popular bakery in the city. And anytime Anne was sent to get the flour needed from the grocery shop, she would hop gladly all the way to there. There were always a lot of people buying, entering, and leaving the large grocery shop and Anne had to wait her turn, so mother always sent her to get the flours very early in the morning when the crowd at the grocery shop consisted of just a few people.

Anne would hurry to the grocery shop gladly and watch Mr.smith, the owner of the grocery shop as he monitored all the workers in the large building, since Anne had to wait her turn she would run over to Mr. Smith and follow him around as he monitored the workers, counted the bags, replaced the tags and eased any difficulties in the grocery shop. Anne felt very proud and mature when she helped out Mr. Smith.

Mr. Smith didn't talk much but when he saw Anne walk into the grocery shop, his kind Emerald eyes would have a bright glow, and his lips under grace an amused smile under all that bushy beard and mustache.

And when Anne hurried over to him eagerly each day and said hello, he would reply with a gentle wave with laugh lines showing by the sides of his eyes as he smiled kindly. Silently they would both begin their monitoring, and accessing of the grocery shop, till it was Anne's turn to take her flour and head home. Mr.smith always made sure he arranged and checked out Anne's order, he never did that for anyone else, you could never see him working at the counter, only monitoring or instructing except when it was Anne's time to check out, and that was when Mr. Smith would step in, arrange the order and wave her a kind goodbye, still smiling as she continued her journey home.

It had become like a ritual each day to help Mr.smith with his store and to hurry back home with all the flours.

She enjoyed her morning chore and looked forward to it each day.

Going to the grocery shop was no longer a chore for Anne it was more like an opportunity for adventure and fun. She loved the walk to the grocery shop because she could see the plants and rare flowers that did not grow in her garden at home. Sometimes she would bend down to uproot a flower so she could smell it and sometimes even take it back home to plant in her garden.

She loved to gaze at the tall trees as she headed to the grocery shop, she would count the branches, enjoy the wind in her hair and smile at the birds who kept singing up ahead, she would wave at them, and sometimes when she was sure no one was looking, she would sing back at them. And together they would make a wonderful harmony and Anne was sure if any audience heard it they would be stunned by it, but for now, she limited her audience to the trees, birds, and the animals that scurried away in the bushes when she began to sing. She would twirl in circles, and hop on the dried leaves, as she sang with the birds.

She would enjoy her wonderful harmony with the birds until she got on the road to the grocery shop, then she would straighten up, stop her singing, take a bow and hear the imaginary applause of her audience of trees, animals, and flowers, before sprinting to the grocery shop.
She enjoyed doing this each day but more than this she enjoyed her little ritual with Mr.smith every day.

Initially, none of the Elvis children wanted the chore of getting the flours but when they saw how Anne's eyes glowed, how bright her color was, and how eager she was to jump, dance, sing and run around after coming back from the grocery shop each day, soon they too began to ask to go to the grocery shop instead of Anne and to leave their present chores. But mother wasn't having it and she made sure everyone did their normal chores.

Anne's siblings tried to bribe her so they could take her chore but she blatantly refused the bribe each time.
And when they asked her why she loved such a boring chore so much, she would shrug and say dreamily,
"It's not something you could easily explain"

Her siblings always just frowned at her and claimed their chores were better than hers anyway.

Yet she always went happily to the grocery shop each day to get mother's flours.

But slowly mother began to notice something weird with the flours and she was greatly confused as to what was going on.
She wanted to tell Anne but she didn't want to bother her, so she simply let her be.

One-day when Anne got to the grocery shop and was working around the shop with Mr. Smith she heard him complain quietly under his breath of how the bags of flours just kept disappearing and how customers kept complaining about it.

Anne was curious to know what Mr.smith was talking about but she saw how the matter greatly disturbed him, so she kept quiet and simply observed him.

Later when it was time for Anne to taker her bags of flour and head home, Mr.Smith asked Anne a question.
"Anne, tell me have you noticed anything weird happening to the bag of flours you buy from my grocery shop?" He asked looking concerned and tired as he checked out Anne's order.
Anne thought for a while and shook her head slowly
"Not that I know of... but I shall ask mother, she should know," Anne said smiling brightly.
"Indeed, you should ask her if she has noticed anything happening to the bag of flours you buy," said Mr. Smith, but still he did not look relieved.

Anne took her bag of flours and headed home but this time she did not run, neither did she sing, she walked slowly back home, pondering what Mr.smith had said about the flours today. She thought and thought but still, she couldn't understand any of it, so she hurried home and told her mother all that had happened at the grocery shop that morning.

When her mother heard she answered,

"Yes indeed, weird things have been happening to the flours but I didn't want to bother you so I kept quiet, I had planned to see Mr.smith myself this weekend and ask him what was going on myself"

"What do you mean mother?" Anne's asked curiously.

"Well some of the bags of flours simply disappear and now I never have enough to bake at the bakery. It's so weird how the flours are complete one moment and the next one bag is missing or the next I'm left with half a bag of flour instead of a full one, and it's all just a big mystery to me, dear Anne" Mother explained as she arranged her baking supplies in the storeroom of the bakery.

Anne frowned

"Do you have any idea what could be the cause?" Anne asked

"I have no idea, and if this is happening to other customers at the grocery shop, Mr. Smith might soon lose all his customers, I really hope he looks into it. It's terrible for business" mother said sighing.

Anne nodded thoughtfully, acknowledging what her mother had said.

All-day all Anne could think of, was the flours and how they disappeared.

What could cause such a thing?

Mr.smith must be very sad.

What a horrible thing to happen.

Anne thought all day.

The next day she hurried to the grocery shop, hoping to hear better news about the flours and also to tell Mr.smith about what mother had said and to buy some bag of flours as was her usual morning chore.

When she got there she found a loud crowd of disgruntled customers, complaining all at once to Mr. Smith and they all looked very angry, Anne simply ordered her flours and hurried home, feeling very sad for the kind and gentle Mr.smith, now he had to face all those angry customers and still he had no idea why his flours kept disappearing.

Anne was worried about this and that evening when her grandmother, came to visit she told her all about her morning chore of buying flours and about the kind Mr.smith and his disappearing bags of flours.

Grandma listened attentively before nodding slowly in understanding when Anne finished.

"I knew something like this would happen, indeed I knew...I just never knew they would be so sneaky..." Grandma said thoughtfully.

"Who? granny, who?

"Oh it's those mischievous little elves, there's a little elve village not far from here and I just heard that they're having a great moonlight party for the elves in a few days" Grandma answered.

"What does that have to do with the flours?" Anne asked

"Well, I believe they've run out of flour to bake for the moonlight party, and instead of buying more, they're sneaking off and stealing flours from this merchant called Mr.smith and all his customers!" Grandma said and she did not look pleased at all.

"What can we do?" Anne asked worriedly.

"Hmmm... well I have some revealing powder in my purse. When you spray it on the flours and repeat a chant that I'll show you, it will reveal the sneaky elves who are hiding around the bags of flours and want to steal them" Grandma said and Anne clapped gleefully.

" The chant is,

Sneaky elves

Sneaky elves

Hiding all around

Make yourself known

For I know your deed

That's the chant and when the elves appear they must be reported to the queen of the elves at once, so they can be punished and will never repeat such rubbish again" said Grandma, handing the revealing powder to Anne.

"Thank you," Anne called out, before hurrying all the way to the grocery shop, when she got there she breathlessly explained all she had learned to Mr.smith and immediately he and all the workers went ahead to repeat the chant and spray the revealing powder over all the grocery and immediately, disgruntled sneaky looking elves appeared all around to the shock of everyone.

Immediately, the elves were arranged in boxes and taken to the village of elves where they were reported to the queen of elves. The elves were punished appropriately and had to pay for every flour they had stolen.
From that time on, no grocery or bag of flour went missing in the grocery shop.

When it was time for the great moonlight feast of elves, the queen of the elves invited Anne and she gladly attended in her beautiful green dress.

Also, Mr.smith gifted the Elvis family a lot of groceries in appreciation, and Anne was always respected anytime she came to pick up her bags of flours as was her daily chore.

And Anne still enjoys the walk to the grocery shop each day and she still holds her wonderful singing with the birds to her audience of trees, animals, and flowers, as she enjoys the wind in her hair and the smell of the wonderful flowers all around.

Thank you for reading and using this book, you have already taken a step towards your relaxation

Best Wishes